HEALTHY AGING

A Wellness Guide To Aging b

Patricia A Cusack

Copyright © Patricia A Cusack 2023. All rights reserved.

No portion of this book may be reproduced in any form without written permission from the author, except as permitted by U.K. copyright law.

First edition 2023

Book Cover designed and created by the Author using Canva.Com. The image of a woman is a model and unrelated to the author and content of the book. The image is taken from a photograph by Jonya of Getty Images from the Canva library of images.

The information and advice contained in this book are based upon the research and the personal and experiences of the author. They are not intended as a substitute for consulting with a healthcare professional. The publisher and author are not responsible for any adverse effects or consequences resulting from the use of any of the suggestions, preparations, or procedures discussed in this book. All matters pertaining to your physical health should be supervised by a healthcare professional. Please consult with your own physician or healthcare specialist regarding the suggestions and recommendations made in this book. The use of this book implies your acceptance of this disclaimer.

The publisher/author has used their best endeavors to ensure that the URLs for external websites referred to in this book are correct and active at the time of publication. However, they have no responsibility for the websites and can make no guarantee that a site will remain live or that the content is or will remain appropriate.

Every effort has been made to trace all copyright holders, but if any have been overlooked the publisher/author apologizes and will be pleased to make the appropriate acknowledgement in any future edition.

Visit the author's website at: patriciacusack.com

Table of Contents

Introduction

Mindset..1

A Healthy Diet is Vital For Longevity................................17

Keep Moving to Live Fully..37

Everything is Connected Being Connected is Everything...51

Sleep Well Stress Less..63

"Nothing is Permanent, Except Change." *The Buddha*........79

Conclusion..91

References..93

Acknowledgements..95

About the Author...96

Thank You..98

For my children, Louise and Dom

and my Son-in-Law, Paul

Introduction

I'm not an expert in any of the fields that I'm including in this book. Nor am I a scientist. As a baby boomer though, I'm now living proof of much of what I recommend as being important to growing older healthily in mind, body and spirit. I offer a wealth of knowledge on how you might achieve the same goal. From the choices we make in our diet and exercise, to the importance of maintaining a positive mindset, I share my own personal journey and the strategies I've used to age healthily. This book originally started life as a series of posts on Instagram. I have an account there to promote my interest in the science of healthy aging, written mainly for women. I found I drew more people to the posts when I had a selfie to accompany the text. However, I hate taking selfies, or photos of myself, so eventually I collated all the information in my posts and put it into a book.

That book became a memoir as it's about my experience of aging. During the first lockdown of the pandemic, I began writing and, when I had finished, I had the manuscript proofread and then sent it to an agent. She contacted me by email, which began: Dear Patrick, so I knew she hadn't read the book. I duly sent the manuscript to another agent and after three months, I gathered she was not going to respond.

So, rather than spend a lot of time hanging about, maybe not even eventually getting taken on by an agent, I decided to publish it myself. Hence this shorter book - I wasn't sure I could cope with the work involved with a full-length manuscript.

Although initially targeting a female audience, I believe that most of the information and recommendations within these pages apply to anyone looking to live their best, healthiest and, therefore, happiest, life. This book is designed for those seeking to improve their health and well-being as they age. Here, you'll find tools and inspiration to embark on your own journey towards a healthy and fulfilled older life, or to enhance the one you are already.

The Secret of Living Well and Long

Eat Half, Walk Double, Laugh Triple and

Love Without Measure.

Tibetan Proverb

1

Mindset

I've always been interested in, and influenced by, scientific research into what keeps us fit and well in body and mind. I was a teenager in the sixties when, for the first time, youthful fashion overshadowed that of the older woman, and this concentration on youth was reflected in so many other areas, including the music of the time. Now we're in the twenty-first century and looking young is still supposed to be the aim for women of all ages as worship of youth remains prevalent.

For me, appearing younger is about staying fit and healthy and moving freely, as well as having a curious and active mind; in fact, avoiding the stereotypical image of the older woman. I believe I'm a good example of what I'm recommending in diet, exercise, mindset, outlook on life etc, that science has backed up. Though I'm not an expert in any of these areas, what I've put into practice has resulted in me reaching my mid-seventies fit and well, looking younger and writing my second book, so - mentally sharp.

Research into what is involved in living a longer than average life without disease has been going on for some time and the conclusions center on several areas: diet, exercise, quality sleep, various levels of social connection, mindset and a sense of purpose. There is much evidence out there to guide us toward and through the older years but it's up to us whether we use the information. In this book, I'm going to look at each of those areas to pull out that which I've found helpful and put into practice.

Thirty years ago, I made two choices which have proved long lasting, positive and beneficial. I was in my early forties and looking for an activity that would keep me strong and flexible; I had played a lot of tennis in my thirties and thought it was time I took up a new physical activity. I had a friend who had been practicing yoga for many years and highly recommended it, so I thought I'd give it a try.

The other choice involved vegetarianism. I'd been considering giving up eating meat for a while for various reasons, including health - science was revealing how a plant-based diet was healthier than a carnivorous one. Other reasons were: the cruelty involved in animal husbandry and world poverty: the grain fed to just one animal over its lifetime would feed many, many more people than the one animal. Reading a Sunday newspaper supplement, which was dedicated to animal husbandry and the cruel way animals were kept prior to slaughter for food, was the deciding factor. I have not deliberately eaten meat since.

Van Gogh sometimes painted flowers in various stages of life to illustrate the truism that nothing is permanent, everything changes. We pick flowers when they are fresh and vibrant in color; as they age, they deteriorate and lose their vitality and appeal until they have to be thrown in the recycling bin.

For us humans, our lives have been extended beyond the traditionally expected threescore years and ten by science and the knowledge of how to be healthy for longer. We don't have to age the way our parents did; we can take control to a certain extent and live a healthy and active life for as long as possible, thanks to scientific research. There is a limit, though, on the lifespan of humans: one new longitudinal research study[1] shows that we could live to be one hundred and fifty - but that's as far as it goes. A progressive loss of resilience would create that limit, researchers concluded.

Anti-ageing is big business; we find it everywhere: in the blurb on beauty products, fashion advice, ads for supplements, exercise videos etc. It's odd how we use the phrase "anti-ageing" which sounds as though we are against aging, as in anti-racism to mean against racism and anti-sexism to refer to being against sexism. What we are really against are the negative effects of aging rather than actual aging, which is a different matter. After all, the alternative to aging is death! Surely, we all want to age healthily and well, so we are actually pro-ageing.

We live our lives according to the choices we have made and to live longer research is informing us we need to choose not to eat food that isn't good for our gut and we need to choose to exercise and get plenty of quality sleep. We have known for a long time that a poor diet is linked to disease, but recent research informs us what we should eat to keep ourselves healthy. In Chapter 2, we look at diet.

The aging process begins the minute we're born, but it's not until middle age that we start to think about later life. It's then that being aware that the choices we make will create a difference in how we age. Part of the established culture of being 'old' is the way older people look. Physically, bodies can become bent as unused muscles lose the strength to hold them up causing people to stoop. There's a road sign placed in areas inhabited by the elderly that has an illustration of a man and a woman, stooped and with walking sticks to alert road users that old people will probably cross this road. This is a stereotypical image which indicates that as people get older, they become less active and their bodies decline as a result, and so this is how society depicts them.

As we approach the age when we consider we are going to be "old" we begin to make changes to our life, sadly often not those recommended by scientists researching aging. We will have a preconceived idea of what "being old" means. This could mean that we think we can now become less active, but eat the amount we usually eat of food that is not actually providing our bodies with the nutrients it needs. Our wardrobe changes to accommodate a growing waistline, and elasticated trousers become a necessity. Moving less affects our muscles and the ability to do what we were able to do before. None of this is helpful to living a long and relatively disease free life, so reframing our mindset to have a more positive image of the older person we want to be is vital.

I found that in my sixties I really turned my thoughts to the future and what aging meant to me because it seemed more of a reality. Once you're over sixty, there's a whole culture of being 'old' that is easy to become absorbed in. We become targets for advertisers online for funerals and companies that draw up wills, we receive leaflets on care homes in the post, articles on fashions and hairstyles for the 'older woman' encourage us to change the way we look. We see pictures in newspapers showing a fifty-year-old female celebrity looking good and the implication is that it's amazing that she looks the way she does at her age, which by today's standards is definitely not old.

It's just accepted that we deteriorate and there is nothing we can do about that but to resign ourselves to our decline. Many, probably most, people succumb to this culture of being 'old', and for my mother's generation, it was the norm. Few trod a different path. It's hard to avoid the traditional route, but it is possible and more and more people are doing it today.

It's not about denying or ignoring our aging; it's about fully taking on board the changes we go through as we progress into late adulthood, with positivity. Yes, our bodies will deteriorate, but we can adjust our fitness regime to always remain fit and able. Loss of function is the real obstacle to enjoying a fully active old age, but if we treat our bodies properly, it doesn't have to happen.

Having a **positive mindset** is beneficial to our health. There's much research going into this. For instance, I was listening to a fascinating podcast on mindset[11] during which we were told of a study into hotel housekeepers who led very busy working lives going up and down stairs constantly, making beds, pushing linen carts, looking after rooms to ensure they were fit for the guests. When these people were questioned about their fitness regime, they said they didn't have time and were quite stressed about that fact. Tests into their physiological makeup showed them to be on the negative side.

They were told that they already had an adequate fitness regime in their job; they were walking, bending, stretching daily when performing their chores. This knowledge had a big impact on their mindset and when they were tested again weeks later, the results were more positive. So nothing had changed except the way these people viewed their jobs and were aware of the amount of exercise they were actually getting. As a result, their health had improved; they lost weight, decreased blood pressure and started feeling better and more confident about themselves and their bodies. They had changed their mindset, and it had benefited their health.

Not only mindset but how we think about ourselves and our age is important for our health. Recent studies have found that those people who think of themselves as being younger than they actually are have a more youthful brain structure and stronger memory than those who feel themselves to be the same age or older than their chronological age. They also walked faster than those who thought themselves as older or their actual age and they were more likely to be involved in regular exercise.

One study[10] identified age as chronological age, which is the number of years we've actually lived; biological age, which is the age our body is showing itself to be in tests, and subjective age, which is the age we think we are and which is predictive of our physical and mental age. I think of myself as ten years younger than I actually am and it's something I naturally do - I don't have to try. To think yourself too young can be counterproductive, apparently because it may give you less ability to adapt to the changes that occur naturally in aging.

In the study, people were asked how old they felt and chose their answer from one of three responses: I'm younger than my actual age; I'm the same as my actual age; I'm older than my actual age. The people that answered that they were younger than their actual age had more positive biological test results than those who felt themselves to be the same age or older.

It was also found that it was not just down to performance but brain scans revealed increased gray matter volume in the areas associated with language, speech and sound. So people who feel younger actually have the structural characteristics of a younger brain. The researchers don't know for sure whether it's the younger brain structure that is affecting the sense of being younger in those with a younger subjective age or whether they are physically and mentally more active and this has created the physical changes in the brain. Those who feel older may have unthinkingly adopted the stereotype of the older adult and become less active and agile, which affects their cognitive abilities. So the saying "you are only as old as you feel" has much truth in it.

The connection between mind and body was always accepted, particularly in the east, and it was the norm in ancient medicinal systems. In the twentieth century, researchers here in the west, studied the complex links between body and mind in their exploration into how depression affects the physical body. The practices of mindfulness, meditation and yoga were found to help not only the mind but the physiological benefits of a calmer mind were discovered to improve overall health. So being positive is good for the mind and body.

Another study found that people who had a positive view of aging lived about seven-and-a-half years longer than those with a negative view, supporting the theory that the mind-body connection is strong. According to yet another study, middle-aged people with no cognitive impairment who had negative views of aging were more likely to have the brain changes associated with Alzheimer's disease.

In contrast, one research result found that those with positive views of aging were resilient and more likely to recover from major health setbacks. Also, researchers found that individuals with great optimism were more likely to live to age eighty-five or over. Optimistic people had an eleven to fifteen percent longer lifespan.

So, forget the negativity about aging; being positive about your life and speaking positively about others is good for the brain and for our sense of self. Treating life as an adventure with new possibilities to be discovered is life enhancing. Remember, you don't lose your sense of humor because you're old; you're old because you've lost your sense of humor.

Five areas of the world where people live very long lives are known as the Blue Zones[2], named by researchers studying longevity. A study involving the residents of all five areas showed a common attribute to living healthily therefore, happily was **a sense of purpose**, a reason to get up every morning. In Loma Linda in California, USA, the community all belonged to the Seventh-day Adventist Church and their shared religion gave them a strong sense of purpose. Okinawa in Japan has each resident with their own individual purpose for living, which they call ikigai; for some it was exercise, for others it was just the pure pleasure of having reached a great age. Costa Rican centenarians have a strong sense of service to others or their family, which they call plan de vida.

Also life enhancing, I found, is living with the purposeful intention of reaching a very old age. Telling yourself you are going to live to be.... (in my case) say, ninety, ninety-five or even a hundred will mean that you have years ahead to be positive about your life and to remain committed to being healthy and active. Then as you approach that age you just move the goalposts. This allows us to live in anticipation and with hope rather than being fearful of the unknown. Of course, you may not reach the age you are aiming for, but you will have spent your last years living life fully with a positive attitude and hope. Don't let your age define you, let your attitude to life be what defines who you are.

Being curious, open to new experiences and accepting, even welcoming, innovation underlies a positive mindset. There are many examples of people achieving their dream in later years because they believed they could. Writers like Laura Inglis Wilder, who wrote Little House on the Prairie, found fame in her sixties with her books; Anna Sewell wrote

Black Beauty in her fifties and she published it when she was 57; Frank McCourt published Angela's Ashes when he was 66; Mary Wesley wrote The Camomile Lawn in her seventies and Peter Roget of Roget's Thesaurus didn't start writing until he was in his sixties. Sir Ranulph Fiennes climbed Mount Everest when he was 65 and pilot Margaret Ringenberg completed the Round-the-World Air Race at the age of 72. One of the greatest achievements of my own life happened when I was 53. After six years of studying while also working, I graduated from the Open University with a 2.1 in Psychology & Social Policy.

Often, as we get older, we have learned much about that on which we have based our opinions and become resistant to new ideas. We become less open to that which is new; others might see us as being set in our ways. Keeping an open mind, testing new ideas against what we already know, and trying new experiences helps us to keep a youthful outlook.

It's easy and tempting to hark back to when we were young as being the best time of our lives. We had the best clothes, the best music, etc. I see it in some of my friends and I feel they are missing out on so much. I know the market is youth orientated and technology is constantly changing, but the trick is not to feel alienated by all this; encompass it; get to know what's happening in the culture and lives of younger people; learn the basics of how to be a part of the online community. Even just learning how to send an email keeps you in touch with others.

One way to keep our brains active is doing '**brain games**'. These are defined as any activity that stimulates your thinking. That includes any games such as crosswords and Scrabble, chess, Sudoku and Bridge. I've always enjoyed stretching my mental faculties by crosswords and later on, Sudoku but in the last few years I've become engrossed in online games. Currently, Wordle is the new craze in word games and I love its daily challenge, along with Quordle, the same word puzzle but with four words rather than one.

Whether these games actually have any long-term benefits for the brain is still being debated in the scientific community. There are studies that do show a delay in dementia or a slowdown in its progress in those who participate, other research has found no connection. However, according to a study in the November 2016 International Psychogeriatrics, certain thinking skills that decline with age may be helped by playing these games, such as processing speed, planning skills, reaction time, decision making and short-term memory.

Learning new skills and doing routine chores in a different way have been found to be good for the brain - try cleaning your teeth with the opposite hand to the one you usually do it with. Taking up a new hobby, learning a new language all challenge the brain and create new neural pathways that prevent atrophy. It's also good for your sense of achievement to learn a new skill, which improves mental health. When was the last time you did something for the first time?

Being proactive about your aging, rather than just letting it happen, is the way to a fitter and healthier old age. It's never too late to make a change to your lifestyle to improve your health and happiness. Just as we plan our finances for a comfortable older age, perhaps investing in our health while we are relatively young should also be seen as a commitment to our quality of life in older age and our longevity.

2
A Healthy Diet is Vital For Longevity

Your body is a temple we are told by health gurus and treating it as such is what we need to be doing for a healthy and long life. We each are the gatekeeper for our body and what we put in, and how much matters to how healthy we are. Over thirty years ago, I gave up eating meat for a variety of reasons, but mainly because of the cruelty involved in its production. Meat actually provides many nutrients, one of which is first class protein, which our bodies very much need to support our muscles and to avoid frailty. Most plants do not contain all the amino acids to create a first class protein. It meant that I had to learn a lot of basics about nutrition to ensure that I didn't miss out on anything important.

I learned that protein can be acquired from plant-based ingredients by combining them. A first class protein comprises nine amino acids and to ensure they are all included in a meal, combining ingredients from various foods containing a few of these amino acids can create the first class protein your body needs. For instance, combining grains and legumes gives you all nine amino acids; this is why beans on toast is such a good, nourishing basic meal - the grain is in the bread and beans are a legume.

Much research has gone into what makes up a healthy diet. Repeatedly, the result is what has come to be known as the **Mediterranean diet**. This is based on the foods eaten around the sunny Mediterranean coast and is mainly plant based with minimal processing and includes: extra virgin olive oil, beans, legumes, whole grains, nuts, berries (raspberries, blackberries, strawberries, blueberries etc), seeds, eggs and some dairy, green salads, fish and a small amount of meat. Not included as part of a regular diet are: sugar, red meat and saturated fats, as well as heavily processed foods, but these may be consumed occasionally.

Beans in particular have been found to be of benefit to healthy aging; black beans, kidney beans, butter beans, chickpeas (garbanzo beans, or chickpeas, are strictly speaking legumes, as are lentils) etc can all be made into appetizing stews and salads to provide fiber and protein. Salmon is an excellent source of protein as well as omega three fatty acids and it's recommended that we eat fish twice a week. Nuts, too, are an excellent provider of protein but high in fat and so should be eaten in small quantities: I have a few on my daily porridge, along with blueberries - and raspberries when they're in season. Pure almond butter (no added sugar or palm oil) is another source of protein, delicious on sourdough toast for breakfast.

Palm oil has been found to have carcinogenic properties and though the food items that contain it won't have much, it's in so many different products that it builds up to an amount that is not good for health. It's also bad for the planet as it is the cause of much deforestation; multinational companies remove natural forests to plant trees that produce palm oil. It's surprising how many food products contain it, as I found when I wanted to buy nut butters and other spreads, so in order to avoid it checking labels is important.

A large-scale study[3] of postmenopausal women in America found that those who acquired their protein through plants had a lower risk of dementia related death and death from cardiovascular disease. Those who ate more processed red meat had a higher risk of dying with dementia than those who consumed other sources of protein. There's some evidence that the older we get, the less responsive we are to protein, so we need to include more of it in our diet to maintain muscle mass and strength. Including a source at every meal helps to reach that goal.

When I was in my early sixties, I began taking a regular fish oil supplement as I was concerned about whether I was getting enough omega-3 in my diet. Having taken that step, it occurred to me I might as well be eating fish, so after much thought and examining of my conscience, I did so.

This caused me to think again about my commitment to not eating meat; after all, you can now buy organic meat where the animals have lived a good life before ending up on your plate. Meat grown from animal cells is a very new concept and involves no cruelty to animals. However, I've remained a staunch non-meat eater but now call myself a pescatarian as I'm eating fish, not without some guilt, I have to say.

The long living people in the Blue Zone regions ate simple food that could well fit into the Mediterranean diet and grew much of it themselves. Tending to their crops helped to keep them active well into old, old age and consuming the healthy fruits of their labor extended their lifespan. Portion size was an important element in the diet of these long living people. In Okinawa, in Japan, where obesity is not a problem, they have a dietary rule of hara hachi bu, which stipulates that you eat until you are eighty percent full. A good rule to live by as maintaining a healthy weight is vital to longevity.

Shortly after the first lockdown due to Covid, I was diagnosed with **pre-diabete**s. I had to learn how to reverse this condition if I didn't want to get full-blown type 2 diabetes. So what is type 2 diabetes? When insufficient insulin is being made by your body, that is when you are likely to get a diagnosis of type 2 diabetes. Insulin is necessary to clear the blood of glucose and turn it into energy via the cells. We get glucose from the carbohydrates we eat and drink. Too much glucose in the blood leads to many problems which become a diagnosis of diabetes, a lifelong illness.

I learned then that different carbohydrates are digested and absorbed at different rates. The **glycemic index (GI)** is a useful tool to tell us the speed at which carbohydrates raise blood sugar levels: quickly, moderately or slowly.

Foods that are digested slowly and release glucose into the bloodstream gradually have a low GI value. These foods are recommended to be the ones we eat most of, as they are the least processed and don't cause a quick rise in blood sugar levels, known as a sugar spike. Sugar spikes can cause us to overeat because the rapid fall in blood sugar can leave us feeling hungry.

The more processed foods are, the higher up the glycemic index they appear. Basically, the glycemic index is a list of foods separated into the three ranges: high, medium and low, indicating the speed at which each food is digested, so we should consume more carbs from the list of low ones. Highly processed foods like, for instance, white bread, white flour, white rice, white sugar have the fiber removed so are made up of simple carbs which are not good for us. Complex carbs are produced from foods with the fiber still intact that make our digestive system work harder, keeping us regular and unblocked.

Whole grains in foods show that they have not had the roughage removed and should be chosen over white alternatives. Porridge oats make a healthy breakfast, but the least processed ones, which are steel-cut and rolled oats, are even healthier. I find rolled oats easier to find (check labels as many oats are flaked which are, therefore, the most processed) and so I have these nearly every morning, with a spoonful of Greek yogurt added for extra protein (sometimes a spoonful of nut butter, too), topped with nuts, seeds and berries.

Other examples of healthy foods and where they sit on the Glycaemic Index: bread with whole grains is not as high as white bread but will have some sugar in its content, as it is made with yeast which is activated by sugar. Sourdough bread is on the lower end of the glycemic index scale, as it isn't made using added yeast or sugar. Brown rice is lower than white rice as it contains fiber and is therefore slower to raise the blood sugar level. Both are now staples in my diet.

As are avocados which nutritionists highly recommend for their fibre, minerals, and vitamins, all of which help to give us a strong immune system. They are calorific, because of their fat content, but it is considered a healthy fat as it is mainly unsaturated. However, if you are trying to lose weight, they should be eaten as part of a calorie-controlled diet. I eat one or two a week. Another so-called "superfood" that I now eat regularly is quinoa (pronounced keenwa); it's considered a grain because it's eaten in the same way, but it is actually a seed. It comes in various colors, the most popular being white; all are rich in nutrients and contain more fiber and protein than other grains. Quinoa is a rare exception in the plant world because it contains all the amino acids to create first class protein. It also has a high antioxidant content compared to other grains.

Since my pre-diabetes diagnosis, I've incorporated more bean and legume recipes into my diet. I have recently resurrected a Vegetarian Shepherd's Pie recipe I've had for a very long time. I used to make this regularly when I first became a vegetarian; my family and I loved it and it never failed to please when I cooked it for guests. Instead of a meat base, it has brown or green lentils with green or yellow split-peas which are simmered for around three quarters of an hour, with an added French onion stock cube to the water for extra flavour. Then sautéed in olive oil: garlic and chopped onion with chopped celery and carrots, combine with the lentil and split pea base and flavor with herbs and pepper. Place this in a dish, add a layer of mashed potatoes and finally, a sprinkling of cheese. Put in a hot oven for about 20 minutes.

The internet is a rich source of recipes and one I'm currently using is a curry made with beans or chickpeas (or both) and or lentils placed in a slow cooker with whatever vegetables I have left over. Sometimes I buy a cauliflower or sweet potatoes specifically for this. Then I add chopped onion and garlic, coconut milk and stock, sprinkle it with spices, usually: turmeric, cumin, paprika, black pepper and curry powder and set it on high for around four hours. I've seen recipes like this where it's set for six hours, but I don't want overly cooked vegetables.

Bean salad is another way I use beans in my repertoire of recipes. I use a combination of various beans as a basis for my salad. I add chopped sun-dried tomatoes, celery, cucumber, anything I have in the fridge (such as chopped feta cheese or chopped, grilled halloumi) or larder, that would be suitable and sprinkle with ground coriander - fresh coriander if I've got it. I drizzle the oil from the sun-dried tomatoes over the bean mixture as a dressing. Delicious with a slice of sourdough bread.

I recently read an article about tinned beans versus dried. It pointed out that tinned beans are actually processed, whereas dried beans are not. It gave me food for thought. Dried beans are cheaper and contain virtually no sodium. They are, however, time consuming in their preparation. Tinned beans are so easy to use but usually have a lot of sodium in the processing. They can be washed thoroughly, which is what I do when I use them, to reduce the amount of sodium left in. You can buy tins of beans with reduced salt. However, I try to keep a stock of both dried and tinned, favoring the dried version as it seems to be the most healthy, but as beans and legumes are so good for you it's worth sometimes making recipes with tins of them, when time is short.

An item of fruit that I have eaten every day for as long as I can remember is an **apple**. For this book, I looked up the nutritional value of one apple, though I've always known that they are good for you. It contains fifty-two calories, is rich in fiber, antioxidants, carbs and sugars (fructose, sucrose and glucose). Despite the high carbs and sugar, it is low on the Glycemic Index so does not cause a sugar spike. I always eat mine after my main meal. I was interested to learn that it also contains quercetin, which is a flavonoid contained in many plant foods and which may have anti-inflammatory and anti-cancer effects. Scientists studying longevity recommend it as a supplement. The old saying that eating an apple a day prevents visits from the doctor may have something in it, as I'm rarely ill. I do love them though; Royal Gala is the species I now enjoy most, as they are not too acidic.

So apples are most probably anti-inflammatory, which is interesting, as we now know that highly processed foods cause inflammation in the gut, which, apparently, is the trigger of all diseases. If we add either stress or antibiotics to the inflammation, then it becomes dangerously high. By avoiding overly processed foods and eating a largely Mediterranean diet with foods below 50 on the GI index, this danger to our health via our digestive system can be avoided.

Inflammation in the body has been extensively studied by scientists in recent years. Basically, it's linked to the immune system. If you have a good, strong immune system, inflammation is unlikely to be a problem. When you have an injury or infection, inflammation will cause the injured area to become red and swollen as chemicals from white blood cells in other parts of your body rush to the affected area to help you heal. In this case, inflammation is a good thing, but sometimes it is triggered when you are stressed, obese or suffer autoimmune disorders. Then, instead of healing, the inflammation persists over time, which can cause chronic illness.

The Mediterranean diet has been found in studies to play an important role in an anti-inflammatory diet; foods such as tomatoes, olive oil, nuts, fatty fish, fruits and berries and leafy green vegetables are recommended to relieve the symptoms of chronic inflammation. At the same time, we are urged to avoid refined carbohydrates, as well as fried foods, sugary drinks, red and processed meats and margarines.

There is a lot of research going on into the impact of the gut on our overall health as more is being learned about it. We know they link good **gut health** to fewer health problems and lower risk of allergies and autoimmune conditions. Apparently, we need a diversity of microbes in our gut to have a healthy digestive system; if we don't, everything else is out of kilter and the resulting inflammation leads to illness and disease. Again, the Mediterranean diet comes up trumps as it contains a variety of foods, which add to the diversity of microbes it creates in our digestive system. Besides plant food, exercise, sleep and the management of stress are important to maintaining a healthy gut.

Eating more fiber and steering clear of highly processed foods are also recommendations to keep your gut in good health and avoiding antibiotics which kill microbes. If antibiotics can't be avoided, then eating foods that increase microbes is the best course of action to protect your gut. These foods include yogurt, not flavored and as natural as possible - I have a spoonful of authentic Greek yogurt on my daily porridge so I'm hoping this is doing my gut health good. Others are fermented foods such as sauerkraut, kimchi, miso, kombucha and many pickles. I believe the jury is out on whether fermented foods actually are good for the gut, but in countries where it is usual to eat this type of food, they find better gut health and less bowel disease.

Fasting is an area being researched for its benefits to aging well. The 5.2 diet has been popular for the last few years. It involves eating normally for five days and then a restricted amount of calories for the other two. It has worked for me and many people swear by it for weight loss. Apparently, though, longer periods of not eating are required to kick-start the process known to be beneficial for longevity. Two or three days or more is what they suggest. There are scientists specializing in longevity research who recommend eating all the necessary calories and nutrition in a reduced time, such as four hours in every twenty-four and there are others who suggest just one meal a day to reap the benefits.

However, I've recently seen one popular doctor on YouTube urge caution on this, as he was not sure that the research into it so far holds up. I do believe though, that Eastern doctors and gurus have been doing this one meal a day for years and they live long lives, apparently. I would always recommend seeing a doctor for anyone wanting to try these unusual fasting methods.

There has been, and continues to be, a great deal of research into the benefits of fasting to help in losing weight. I reversed my diagnosis of pre-diabetes with the 5.2 diet as I had successfully used it before to lose weight and applied it again to lose the extra pounds I had accumulated over lockdown. I also cut out any highly processed foods, like biscuits, which I was eating way too much of to satisfy the increased hunger that is a symptom of pre-diabetes, and additionally increased the amount of exercise I was getting. It was a relief to learn eventually that I was out of the danger zone and type 2 diabetes was no longer a threat. I have since learned that I have a gene that gives me an increased risk of the disease, so I have to be careful it doesn't happen again.

I am currently eating all my calories in a six-hour time slot, starting with breakfast between eight and nine o'clock and then lunch between two and three o'clock. I've found this to suit me very well as, by bedtime, my digestive system is about ready to rest, along with the other parts of my body. Maintaining this regime means I am effectively fasting for a large part of each day. To help me with this, I use an app installed on my iPad where I have established how many calories I need to consume and then I log my food for the day. The app informs me of the nutritional value of what I'm eating and how many calories I've eaten.

There are scientists who recommend longer periods of fasting occasionally, say twenty-four to forty-eight hours or even longer once a month or every three months. I haven't yet tried that. The science behind this is that long periods of food abstinence triggers autophagy, which is the process of removing damaged cells, helping the body to cleanse itself. This stimulates the production of growth hormones. Autophagy is considered a crucial defense mechanism against infections and other damaging malignancies. It's part of a cell's natural lifecycle and is essential to keep your immune system free of disease.

However, exposure to chemicals, stress and aging can damage our cells, which leads to inflammation and the accumulation of toxins. Intermittent fasting of, say, sixteen hours every night can trigger autophagy but longer periods may produce more effective results. This is not recommended without discussing the process with your doctor.

Almost every day I read something in my news app about research into aging. We are learning more and more about how to live a healthy life via science so that we can live a longer life that is free from illness. There are several components that go into this healthy life we should live and diet and exercise are two that are frequently researched by scientists from various angles. Sometimes, findings conflict with the accepted results from previous research, as, for instance, with **supplements**; a multivitamin was thought the way to go when our diet might be lacking for some reason, such as vegetarianism or aging digestive systems that weren't working efficiently. Then it was found in some studies that those taking a multivitamin were not living as long as those who weren't, so now we're advised not to take a multivitamin but to take individual vitamins and minerals, according to our needs.. I started taking a daily multivitamin when I gave up eating meat. As a result of the change of advice I now take various supplements where I think I may be lacking.

I was listening to a podcast on hormones and the subject of the immune system was discussed by the medical practitioners. The topic of Supplements was introduced and how important it is to keep the immune system strong. It was recommended to take: Zinc, Magnesium and Vitamin D to help strengthen the immune system and I was pleased to realize that I do already take those supplements. As the Covid pandemic got underway, there was talk about Vitamin D being essential to the immune system to fight the impact of the illness. There seemed to be an online debate about this for a while, but I think the proponents won the argument.

A glass of wine or a cold beer can be a welcome addition to a meal or to just relax when socializing with friends. What does science tell us about consuming **alcohol**? Is it good for us or to be avoided? The results of a large-scale research study a few years back told us it's better to have some alcohol than none at all - the people in the study who drank some alcohol did better than those who abstained in health tests. Scientists put it down to the resveratrol in the wine that most of them drank and the ingredient became a source of study in itself with regards to longevity. Resveratrol is a natural ingredient found in the skin of red grapes, so red wine became the popular choice for those health-conscious people who are partial to alcohol.

Drinking alcohol is still considered a cancer risk, particularly if consumed in large quantities, but the occasional tipple, especially if imbibed with food, is supposedly safer than drinking the recommended amount.

Smoothies are a recent phenomenon and one which I have happily embraced. They are not only delicious but very healthy, allowing you to consume more fruit and vegetables. As we age, our digestive systems become less efficient and, for me, a morning smoothie ensures I am getting the extra nutrition I need. The juicer required to mix the fruit and vegetables is a small kitchen gadget that doesn't take up much room. Since having been gifted one as a birthday present by my health conscious son, I've used it daily and I'm consuming more spinach & kale (both of which contain lutein which is good for the eyes), celery, chopped root ginger, carrots, raw beetroot and sometimes oat or nut milk. I place an avocado in my daily smoothie twice a week, which makes a rich mousse-like consistency and is delicious. I also add a protein powder to help ensure I get sufficient protein. I'm still experimenting with it.

We have to be aware that smoothies could be unhealthy if too many fruits are used, and sugar or honey added. Keeping the sugar levels down in my diet is important because of my previous pre-diabetes diagnosis, so I'm very conscientious about this. I've also read a couple of articles by a dietician and a scientist which were both negative about smoothies, in that the process of chopping up the vegetables to a pulp removes the fiber; the fiber being an important ingredient in the nutritional makeup of the food. However, on weighing up the pros and cons, I've decided that consuming extra green vegetables this way and the nutrients they provide, is a definite benefit to health. The secret is to not pulverize the vegetables but to leave some fiber intact with a textured consistency rather than an entirely smooth constituency.

Changing your diet may seem a drastic step if you're used to eating the meat and two veg regime that we inherited from our predecessors. Eating this way wasn't always so. It began with the agricultural revolution and the ready availability of food. Unfortunately, we now have too much availability with a boom in the number of takeaway food outlets and eateries. This food is not usually healthy and obesity is becoming a tremendous problem. Knowing that too much food and certainly too much processed food can cause disease, we have the choice of taking control of our aging process by eating only that which is good for us and in smaller portions.

Another element in healthy aging is activity - keep moving to stay healthy and strong. More on this in the next chapter.

3
Keep Moving to Live Fully

Besides eating healthily and having a positive mindset, exercise is another vital component in aging well. Scientific research has shown us that the people who continue to be active as they age live longer than those who don't. Slumping in front of daytime television is definitely not recommended for those who want to go into their latter years, fit and well. We have a choice of how we treat our bodies and if we choose to keep them flexible and strong with efficient digestive systems, we should be in a better position to repel illness and or to cope with it.

When I took up **yoga** over thirty years ago, little did I know it would be one of the best investments I would make for my older years. I'm still practicing it but via Zoom rather than attending live classes. My teacher, Jules, took her classes online during the first lockdown in 2020 and still offers that choice. It suits me to do it that way after my diagnosis of ocular hypertension in both eyes four years ago, which is a **pre-glaucoma** condition. According to the NHS website, glaucoma is a common eye condition. The optic nerve becomes damaged; this nerve connects the eye to the brain. It's usually caused by fluid building up, which increases pressure inside the eye. The condition can lead to loss of vision if not diagnosed and treated early [9].

My paternal grandmother, Granny Rose, was diagnosed with glaucoma when she was 70 and, as there was then nothing to prevent blindness from the condition, that was her eventual fate. Science has since developed eye drops, which, if used regularly, will keep full blown glaucoma at bay. Fortunately, if I continue to use the eye drops every day for the rest of my life, I will, hopefully, have a different fate from my Granny Rose.

I learned from a research study that certain yoga asanas, or poses, can increase the hypertension in the eyes so I substitute them where possible or ensure I don't hold the postures for very long. The asanas to avoid are inverted postures, such as Downward Facing Dog (*Adho Mukha Svanasana*) - I do the Plank (*Kumbhakasana*) pose instead, Legs Up the Wall (*Vipanta Karani*), the Plough (*Halasana*) and forward bending poses. If I attended an actual class, I feel it may disconcert other yoga students to see me not following instructions, so Zoom classes are perfect for my situation.

Over thirty years of practicing yoga has helped in so many ways, besides the fitness aspect. I will never be so flexible that I can place my limbs into unbelievable contortions, but I think I must be more flexible than if I had never taken it up. I had a break from practicing for a few years during my fifties; when I took it up again, it shocked me how difficult just getting down to the floor and getting up again had become. Regular yoga makes you so agile and fit that you don't realize what you'd be like if you weren't doing it. As we age, our joints begin to stiffen and regular yoga can help reduce joint stiffness. It also helps with balance, can reduce stress and improve blood flow.

We now know that being able to get up from the floor adds years to your life. Practicing yoga means that you retain that ability. Research has found that those people who can get up from the floor without using their hands are more likely to be alive in six years' time. Continually sitting in chairs results in weak leg muscles. In Japan they sit on very low seats, so getting up and down activates leg muscles that sitting on higher chairs doesn't bring into use. Can you get up from your chair without using your hands? This is a good measure of the strength of your leg muscles and doing it regularly helps to activate them.

Another method to try is to kneel on the ground (on something soft to protect your knees) in a high kneeling position; put your left foot forward and place it on the ground. Without using your hands, push up onto that leg into a standing position and bring the right leg alongside it. Then reverse the process - put your right leg back and place the knee on the knee protection, bringing the other knee alongside it. Put your right foot forward and place it on the ground; without using your hands, push up onto that leg and bring the other alongside it. You may need to press your hands onto your thigh when you first start practicing this, but as your legs strengthen, you should be able to do it without using your hands.

The twenty-first century is changing the shape of the human body in that modern technology is requiring us to hold our heads down and forward to read the screens of our computers, phones and iPads, pushing our head out of alignment with our spine. This can become a painful position and should be corrected. Regular yoga makes you aware of your body, so that your posture improves. When you're standing in a queue or sitting at a desk, you become aware of how you are standing or sitting and can ensure that your body is realigned, which is good for your skeleton. Think of a piece of string attached to the top of your head and someone pulling it up. This makes you stand tall.

As a regular practitioner of Hatha Yoga, you learn about breathing, how controlling the breath helps with stress - breathing in deeply and slowly, then out deeply and slowly several times calms a tense body.

Yoga is one of the six schools of Hinduism and has been practiced for centuries, but science backs up claims that it is good for you and slows aging. The word "Yoga" is from the Sanskrit and means to unite, as in the body and the mind. Researchers have shown in studies that it helps to reduce stress, which can be dangerous if not treated. One study indicated that performing yoga postures, breathing techniques and meditating for three months actually slowed the aging of the cells. So, if it does that after three months, how much more benefit and improvement in longevity is practicing it for a lifetime?

Another exercise regime I started during lockdown I found on YouTube: **Qi gong**. Like yoga, qi gong started in the east as a spiritual pathway, but in the west is looked upon as an exercise regime. However, it also uses breathing techniques and practitioners view it as a mind and body practice. There are two Buddhist monks I follow along with as they show how to perfect this ancient system. They both wear the traditional garb which I love to see.

Walking is another activity that I've always chosen to do when possible and during the first lockdown, I walked most days and still try to take two or three long walks a week. Studies have shown that brisk walking is particularly beneficial to the heart. It can lower the risk of high cholesterol, high blood pressure and diabetes. From my own experience, it also seems to help my knees in that, if I have periods of not walking for some reason, one of my knees is painful. Researchers from multiple studies found that walking reduced the risk of heart disease by 31% and cut the risk of dying by 32%. These results were found in both men and women in the studies.

Regular walking also helps with fat loss, maintains muscle mass and bone density too. I know a few people who are over ninety and most of them walk daily. Walking in the countryside improves our sense of wellbeing and I am lucky where I live to be able to do that. In cities, parks provide excellent places for regular walking and running.

It's long been advised to aim for 10,000 steps a day for the optimum benefit of walking to protect against dementia, heart disease and cancer. However, a new study[4] has concluded that walking speed is more important than the number of steps. There's no denying that achieving 10,000 steps a day reaps substantial rewards for your health, but this study demonstrated that walking 3,800 steps at a faster rate can cut the risk of dementia by 25 percent. So brisk walking or power walking can be beneficial too if you can't make the 10,000 steps every day. In fact, the research showed that every 2,000 steps walked reduced the risk of premature death by 8 - 11%. The more steps walked reduces the risk of dementia.

There's no reason older people shouldn't run as that, too, is good for muscle strength and heart health. Walking may be more sustainable for older people compared to **running** but I have friends who are in their late seventies and eighties who take part in park runs, which are organized events for anyone who wants to compete with others of their age and provides a good incentive to keep running. It enables them to achieve twice as much exercise as walking because they do more in the same amount of time. **Cycling**, too, is good for the leg muscles and I have an exercise bike for the days when I can't get out for whatever reason.

Walking, running and cycling build stamina but we also need other types of exercise for all round fitness. After middle-age adults lose 3% of their muscle strength every year, so as we age our muscles become weaker and if we do nothing we can develop **sarcopenia**, which is a condition of age-associated muscle degeneration, common in people over fifty. If this happens, we lose the ability to do much of what we were used to doing.

Bones are held together by ligaments which attach the muscles to the bones, so it's important to have strong muscles. If an elderly person falls, they need to be able to get back up. **Weight training** is important to maintain independence. It also helps strengthen bones. It's never too late to start. Weights and resistance bands are an essential part of the exercise regime of the over fifties. Building and maintaining muscle mass is vital and regular practice with these aids will ensure strength is upheld.

Squats are a leg exercise which has many benefits: they improve bone density thereby preventing osteoporosis; burn fat, protect the knees by strengthening the muscles there and increase flexibility in the leg joints and hips. When I learned this, I incorporated squats into my weekly regime. Sometimes I do them as a part of a sequence, other times I will just get up and do ten or multiples of ten squats, which stretches my legs and back after lengthy periods of sitting at the computer.

Aerobic exercise is excellent for heart health and that means any regular movement that gets the heart working harder. Within the last few years, **HIIT** has been shown by researchers to have huge benefits to people of all ages. The acronym HIIT stands for High-Intensity Interval Training. It's a training technique that allows you to accomplish high intensity training in a short period of time. I try to incorporate this into my weekly exercise routine once a week. I have five exercises I use, which are: running hard on the spot; touching alternate knee to elbow as fast as possible; star jumps, squats and jumping on the spot. Each exercise is carried out in short bursts of 30 seconds, then rest for 10 seconds, so a stopwatch or a means of gauging time is essential. The set of exercises is then repeated as many times as you are able. The sequence can also be carried out on an exercise bike or other machine, with short bursts of rapid cycling, then rests, then short bursts of rapid cycling, etc.

One of the most important components of a fit body is healthy lungs. Breathing in through the nose is important as the nasal passages cleanse the air of impurities which is missed by breathing in through the mouth. So unless you're having to breathe hard during an arduous workout it's best to try to always breathe through the nose. The air then goes into our lungs and travels into our blood vessels, oxygenating the blood, which then goes to the heart where it is pumped to the rest of the body.

For smokers, the smoke they inhale destroys lung tissue by leaving a coating of tar from the nicotine, which prevents oxygen from the air they breathe reaching the blood vessels. Over time, lack of oxygen has a devastating impact on the body. Smoking has been found to be a prominent cause of lung cancer and anyone wanting to age healthily is advised to not go there. During my youth everyone smoked and during the sixties I did too. I took it up in my teens to be part of the "in crowd". However, after about four years, I gave it up and hopefully did no lasting damage to my health.

One eminent longevity researcher makes the suggestion that our bodies are used to the stress caused by adverse conditions and research has shown that some stress does us good; the overly heated lifestyle we have become acclimated to today isn't healthy, apparently. One way to "healthily" stress our body is through cold showers. The shock of the cold water gives a slight boost to the immune system and activates the sympathetic nervous systems which governs the fight-or-flight response in frightening or dangerous situations. A study has shown that it improves circulation. However, there are some risks to immersion in cold water, especially for people with heart conditions. In older adults, cold water applied just to the neck and face area has been shown to improve brain function, apparently and has been used to help combat dementia.

Several studies have looked at people in middle-age and the effects of physical exercise on their thinking and memory in later life. One particular study[5] looked at health behaviors of over 2,000 men in Wales and followed them for thirty- five years. Five behaviors were assessed: regular exercise, not smoking, moderate alcohol intake, healthy body weight and healthy diet. Exercise was found to have had the greatest impact in reducing the dementia risk. There was a sixty percent reduced risk of developing dementia by people who followed four or five of the assessed behaviors.

The healthy lifestyle necessary to achieve a disease free life was down to five habits: eating healthily, regular exercise, keeping a healthy body weight, not smoking and moderate drinking. Researchers found that women who practiced four of the five healthy habits at the age of fifty lived an average of 34.4 more years free of diabetes, cardiovascular diseases and cancer, compared to 23.7 healthy years in women who practiced none of these healthy habits. Men who practiced four out of five of the healthy habits at the age of fifty were found to live 31.1 years free of chronic disease compared to 23.5 years amongst men who practiced none.

Less research has been done on healthy older people, but there is evidence to show that they can also reduce their risk of dementia with regular exercise, especially aerobic exercise. An active daily life which includes brisk walking, cleaning or gardening can be included in this.

So it's about what we do with our bodies; what we put into them and how we keep them active that is important to our experience of old age. We are conditioned to like sweet things from our youth, but cutting back on sugar and salt is important to our health, this and other studies have found. Exercising around 30 minutes a day and keeping our weight within the BMI guidelines is recommended, as well as not sitting for long periods of time. With regard to exercise, YouTube has an enormous volume of videos from a variety of sources on exercise: yoga, qi gong, walking on the spot, running on the spot, weight training, Pilates, HIIT, etc., etc. During lockdown, I found innumerable useful videos to add to my playlist to help keep me fit and flexible.

It takes commitment and discipline with diet and exercise to maintain a healthy lifestyle. In fact, adopting a whole new mindset is necessary: refusing the daily biscuit with coffee, reducing the portions of food we're used to, moving more and ensuring we incorporate the various aspects of exercise into our routine. However, the rewards are well worth the effort.

In the next chapter, we look at the importance of human connection through relationships for a long and relatively disease free life.

4
Everything is Connected Being Connected is Everything

Researchers into longevity have found that five levels of social connection were experienced by those who lived the longest lives and they are: spouse or partner, family, friends, wider social circle and shared belief system or worldview. To have four of the five levels of connection is still considered to be of benefit to longevity.

Being in a **long term committed relationship** is definitely good for your physical and mental health, studies show. Single people who have good social support can also be happy, and those who decide to leave an unhappy marriage can find happiness if they have sound support. What about men's and women's different lived experiences of marriage or long-term commitment? Are they similar? Research reveals that for men it's definitely a positive to be married. A major study in America found that married men are healthier than those who don't marry or whose marriages end in divorce or widowhood. They live longer than men who don't marry and the longer they are married, the greater their survival chances are than those who are unmarried.

I've heard it said that men should marry an educated woman if they want a long life and the results of research have shown that there is some truth in this. There are studies that show that men whose wives were well educated had lower risks of a plethora of adverse health conditions and overall a lower death rate than those whose wives were less well educated. Maybe this is because more educated women learn how to take responsibility for their own health and, consequently, that of their husband's.

Another factor is loneliness. Having a wife staves off this potentially deadly condition. Unmarried people who live with a partner tend to show better outcomes in studies than those living alone, but for men living with a wife they enjoy the best of all health. Research into bereavement shows that men are more likely than women to experience illness and disability after losing a spouse. It seems that having been looked after by their wife and before that, their mother, they become unable to look after their own nutritional needs and their overall health, although grief itself can debilitate, resulting in loneliness, depression and social isolation.

Studies make clear that men would enjoy more positive outcomes if they took control of their own health, especially when single. Research shows that unmarried, divorced and widowed men don't eat well or exercise and are more likely to engage in unhealthy behaviours such as smoking and drinking alcohol. So, if marriage benefits men more than women, I wondered what science says about women and wedlock.

Women have long been more unhappy with the marital state than men. Studies show that around seventy percent of divorces are initiated by women. It was not so long ago that society frowned on divorce and unhappy couples stayed together for the sake of avoiding social ostracism and the costs involved, especially for women who were not encouraged to work outside the home. Today, women are more likely to work and can be self-supporting. It's not always easy, but it can be done. Also, divorce has become part of the norm, so leaving a marriage does not mean social alienation.

The sorts of behavior women were expected to accept by their spouses is no longer tolerated. Men are more likely to commit adultery and engage in risky behavior. It has been mooted that women have high expectations of marriage and are too soon to act when it doesn't live up to their expectations. Perhaps the finding of "the one" still lingers in a girl's upbringing, judging by the popularity of the number of fairy tale weddings that still take place.

There's no question that men and women are socialized differently. Men have been brought up to concentrate on their own needs and to consider material contributions more important, as they still expect to be the breadwinner. Women, in contrast, are raised to put the needs of others first and to prioritize empathy and caring. This can lead to a conflict of expectations. When "Mr Right" doesn't turn out to be as helpful around the home as a woman expects and lacks understanding of his wife's annoyance at this, problems arise in the relationship. Marriage definitely means compromise for both partners, but more women are coming to the conclusion that it's no longer worth the sacrifices required of them.

The Office for National Statistics in the UK[6] reveals from censuses that marriage and divorce are on the rise at age sixty-five and over. The number of older people getting married went up by forty-six percent in a decade. This has been attributed to the post-war baby boomers making up twenty percent of the population and they are living longer. Almost all the brides and grooms aged over sixty-five in 2014 were divorcees, widows, or widowers, and only eight percent were getting married for the first time.

The studies that show that the longest living people have five levels of connection indicate that staying married when the relationship is good is worth it for both parties when it comes to longevity. However, for the women who leave unhappy marriages, at whatever age, they can still find happiness through their network of friends. Women are better at maintaining their friendships, even during marriage, than men, and this can be a crucial factor in their health and wellbeing after the loss of a spouse. I can vouch for this as I left a marriage in my early seventies and now live happily without a life partner, surrounded by not only friends, but a close family.

The next level of connectedness in the studies into longevity was to **family**. Those people who had close family members were found to live longer than those who didn't.

The long living people in the Blue Zone regions lived either with, or very close to, family members and there were no retirement homes in the vicinity. The mixing of different generations would be good for all concerned, and interactions with young people would be stimulating for the elderly family members, giving them a strong sense of connection to life.

Perhaps until the middle of the twentieth century the trend was towards single-family homes. However, the number of multi-generational living arrangements in the UK and the US, as well as other developed countries is growing. With women working and childcare costs high, the help of grandparents is essential. That and the fact that fewer young people just can't afford to live independently means that they have little choice but to continue living with their parents. So both generations involved are experiencing several benefits: financial, psychological and social. The older members of these families have been shown in studies to have a longer survival rate than those living on their own.

The third level of important connectedness for longevity is that of **friends.** Having a network of good supportive friends is vital at any age, but particularly in later years, especially if you live alone. The quality of the relationships you have with friends is essential and often developed over time. The quantity is irrelevant if the few that you have are real and with whom you can be yourself. You may have hundreds of Facebook and Twitter "friends" but they don't count when it comes to quality. These superficial social media connections can lead to a feeling of insecurity and exacerbate loneliness.

Nurturing your relationships with close friends is important for your mental health. It has been said that friends are the family we choose instead of being born into. Close friends provide unconditional love that not all families share. They stand by you regardless of what you're going through and they are always there for you, offering support and inspiration, sometimes supplying a reality check in a situation we are not seeing clearly. Good friends support your dreams and goals and encourage you to achieve them.

In Japan the residents have friendship groups of five people who commit to each other throughout their lives; these groups are called Moais. They were originally formed for financial reasons but eventually became mutual support networks. Women in any country are more likely to have such a friendship group, or **Moai**, which might be part of the explanation for them living longer than men. Living alone means that my own circle of friends is invaluable and I cherish each one. We are nearly all online and email or phone each other but ensure that we meet regularly in person at least monthly.

However, hanging on to friendships when they no longer supply the support you need but cause you to be unhappy is no longer productive in your life. It's better to face up to the fact that it's time to call it a day. No longer enjoying a friendship can lead to stressful situations which can be detrimental to your mental, and consequently, physical health.

Next, and fourth, in the levels of connection is a **wider social circle,** as found in activity groups and they are often where new friends are made. The groups might be arts and crafts sessions, sports groups, book clubs, writing circles, knitting circles, keep fit groups, yoga, Pilates, choirs, study groups for those who like to continue to learn as they age, etc. Over the years, I have been a member of many of these and I've made most of my friends through them.

We get to know more people through activity groups and enjoy the social interaction even though they are not on the same level of intimacy as our close friends. We share a familiarity and a common experience in the group's activity. Over time, one or two of these people may join our inner circle of friends. For those that don't, their very familiarity can make us feel part of a community. They help us feel rooted.

The final connection level is a **shared worldview, belief or religion**. Every culture on earth gathers in social groups; it's a natural human instinct to do so. The long living peoples studied for their longevity usually enjoyed being part of a religious community. The feeling of connection in such a community must be life enhancing. As someone who is not religious, I see the activities enacted in the churches as the glue for the communities, rather than the religion itself. The congregations meet regularly; they sing and pray together, often they provide support networks as well as social networks and they share a set of common beliefs.

Some of the other groups mentioned earlier fulfill the roles provided by churches: regular meetings, sharing group activities and common beliefs. Contributing to society in whatever way we can, such as volunteering (for me, fourteen years of volunteer counseling and getting library books for the elderly and housebound, as well as a short time helping in a food bank) or political activism - even armchair activism, encourages a sense of involvement and self-worth, which achieves something that can positively affect others.

Another important relationship is the one we have with our **pets**. There is research that shows the benefit of owning a pet at any age. Pet ownership has grown hugely since the beginning of the pandemic. When Covid forced lockdown on societies, rather than face life alone, people obtained pets, particularly dogs. The dog, apparently, is the oldest domestic animal, sharing their lives with humans for nearly ten thousand years with evidence from tomb paintings, artefacts and texts revealing that people at all levels of society have kept them as pets.

Studies show that physical contact with a beloved pet is very beneficial to the owner, helping to lower stress levels and making them feel happier and less lonely. Also, the bond that is created by the nurturing and caring for a dog is beneficial to both pet and owner, the dog has all its needs met by its "human". This has created a vast market in dog related accessory sales as they are treated more like miniature humans than animals with, as well as food, bedding and vets' bills, toys and clothes being marketed and bought by caring dog owners.

The result of one piece of research into pet ownership I found surprising; when studying the demographics of pet ownership, researchers found that older people were less likely to have a dog or a cat. According to participants in the Baltimore Longitudinal Study in the USA, pet ownership was lower in people of older decades. However, pet ownership has shown to be better for improving cognitive and physical function and generally seems to be good for the owners.

According to a survey in the UK thirty-three percent of people owned dogs while twenty-seven percent were cat owners. Another piece of research tells us that owning a cat is better for your carbon footprint as the resources needed to feed it over its lifetime is not as much as that of a dog because cats eat less and are more likely to eat fish based food than corn or beef products. A study in the UK in 2010 found that people who owned cats were more likely to have a college degree than dog owners Another study in Wisconsin concluded that cat owners were more intelligent but the researchers carrying out the Bristol University study in the UK said that it's because smarter people tend to work longer hours and cats need less attention than dogs.

Having five levels of connectedness, then, is important for longevity. Enjoying some sense of being involved with others and feeling fulfilled can dispense with loneliness. Being alone and being lonely are two very different situations and to feel lonely is not good for our health; the stress of loneliness can cause insomnia and depression. Getting good sleep and knowing how to cope with stress can help our mental health and that is what we discuss in the next chapter.

5
Sleep Well Stress Less

Another important element in healthy aging is getting enough **sleep**. Adequate sleep is important for our sense of well-being, physically and mentally. Poor sleep affects the hormones that regulate appetite and has been shown to impair brain function. It can also lead to pre-diabetes because of the adverse effects on blood sugar levels; perhaps this was one of the causes that contributed to my own diagnosis of pre-diabetes; I was not sleeping well due to the circumstances enforced by lockdown during the beginning of the pandemic.

There is a great deal of research going on into sleep: how much we need, the conditions which are best for optimal sleep, supplements that can help with sounder sleep, etc. Regularly getting poor quality sleep is being recognised as putting us at serious risk of developing medical conditions affecting longevity. The NHS recommends we get around eight hours of good sleep a night; some will need more, some will need less, but getting uninterrupted deep rest is vital for long-term health.

The conditions needed to get good quality sleep are:

– Avoid eating a large meal or consume caffeine before bedtime,

– Put the screens away an hour before retiring,

– Have rosemary or lavender in some form in your room,

– Ensure the pillows and covers are comfortable,

– and that the bedroom is dark, cool and quiet.

– If you're a reader, then a chapter of your current book will induce drowsiness.

If sleep still evades you there are several exercises to try such as deep breathing: inhale to the count of 8, hold the breath to the count of 4, exhale to the count of 8 and hold to the count of 4, repeat three or four times. Another breathing exercise is box breathing where you breathe in to the count of 4, hold to the count of 4, breathe out to the count of 4 and hold the count of 4, then repeat several times. Or a counting exercise: count two parallel rows of numbers at the same time, starting with 1 then 15, then 2, then 14, 3, 13 and so on until you complete each row; the concentration involved in this exercise should send you to sleep!

Recent research into the role of sleep in our immune system[12] tells us that as long as we get good quality sleep, the amount is not as important as was once believed. Those people in a study who had less sleep than the recommended amount and reported that it was poor quality suffered more colds and flu in the ensuing weeks than those who reported having slept well but still had fewer hours of sleep. This is reassuring to people who have no choice but to sleep restricted hours because of their jobs and to those who don't achieve the recommended amount but still get some good quality sleep.

Taking an **afternoon nap** can help to cope with extreme tiredness when you're not sleeping well. However, I've always tried to have a zizz when my energy levels slump after lunch. It's not always possible, but it definitely gives me an energy boost when I do. The benefits of napping have been recognized by many companies who want their employees to stay energetic and alert in the afternoon. In Japan, the practice is becoming very popular in workplaces. Apparently, Google offers their employees dark, soundproof booths to power nap in.

The Spanish have the siesta incorporated into their daily lives and studies show that it is a very healthy thing to do. It has been found to relax the heart and reduce stress, increase mental response, enhance alertness and improve digestion. As long as the nap doesn't become a long sleep, research shows that it helps the completion of sleep cycles.

Researchers studied a cohort of 23,000 Greek adults[7] for an average of six years and found that occasional napping decreased a person's risk for heart disease by 12%, but regular napping decreased the risk by a huge 37 percent. However, napping is not recommended for people who suffer from insomnia, as it may interfere with attempts to re-establish a bedtime routine, making you less tired when it's time to sleep.

Coping with **stress** is very important for mental and physical health. We can't control what life throws at us to deal with, but we can learn how to get through the adverse situations by reducing the stress they create in our bodies and minds. It's particularly important in our later years that our stress levels are kept to a minimum as science is showing us that chronic levels of stress at any age but particularly in later years, can lead to serious illnesses.

We also now know through scientific research that when we get stressed, the telomeres, which are caps on the end of chromosomes, shorten and thus reduce length of life. Older women have been proven to be especially susceptible to producing too much cortisol, which is a stress hormone. Producing too much cortisol has been linked to many health problems and adversely affects the storage retrieval of memories. If chronic stress is not reduced over a long amount of time it could result in Alzheimers.

The importance of **breathing practice** has long been recognised by eastern traditions, yoga being one of them with its branch of Pranayama, which is breath yoga. We are now recognising how controlling the breath helps reduce stress. For me, learning breathing exercises via yoga was a tremendous help in controlling my nerves before I had to undergo something I considered stressful. The first one I learned in a yoga class was this (similar to the one I use sometimes to help to get back to sleep mentioned earlier):

– Breath in deeply counting to 8

– Hold and count to 4

– Breath out counting to 8 - this is the most important part of the exercise to calm everything down so don't rush it.

– Hold and count to 4

– Do the above for 5 breaths.

To do it correctly you need to be sitting up straight but I found that wherever I was, perhaps standing outside a door waiting to go in and undergo some very stressful procedure, it helped to just do this simple breathing exercise. It calms the system down, which in turn calms the mind; it's all interconnected.

We tend not to think about breathing usually. We just do it unthinkingly and because of this our breathing can be shallow - the breath goes no further down than the chest so our blood is not being properly oxygenated. When our blood cells take in oxygen, carbon dioxide is released, which we then exhale. If this process is being hampered by incorrect breathing, in potentially stressful situations, it can signal a stress response. Breathing deeply in and down into the stomach (you should feel it extending as it fills with air) activates your nervous system, which relaxes the body and helps you to avoid the fight-or-flight response we experience in a stressful situation.

Breathing through the nose rather than the mouth is also important and helps to oxygenate our blood. When exercising, it is sometimes difficult to breathe through the nose because of the intensity of the breath and then breathing through the mouth is the only way. However, those who normally breathe through the mouth are doing their health a disservice. It leads to sleep apnoea, which disturbs sleep and it then follows that disturbed sleep becomes the norm, and this can lead to serious health issues.

Alternate nostril breathing is another deep breathing exercise I learned through yoga. It's a good way to relieve tension and be present in the moment. For this, you need to be seated comfortably, sitting with a straight spine (imagine the string being pulled up out of the top of your head). Rest your left hand in your lap, then with your right hand:

Place the index and middle fingers centrally between your eyebrows (the spot known as the "third eye" in yoga), press your thumb into the right nostril, closing it off then breathe in through the left nostril. Close off your left nostril with your third finger whilst holding the breath, then breathe out through the right nostril. Breathe in through the right nostril, then closing it off with your thumb, breathe out through your left nostril. Breathe in through the left nostril, then closing it off with your ring finger, breathe out through your right nostril. Repeat this sequence several times, starting off with, say, three or four, working up to about ten rounds. If you feel light-headed at any point, stop and breathe normally.

Another useful practice to help stress, taken from eastern philosophies, is **meditation**. Learning to sit quietly every day for however long you are able can give a feeling of calmness when you are living in some turmoil. Meditation is scientifically backed and there are various methods you can try to find your favorite way to achieve a state of calm and a peaceful mind. Mentally following the breath as you inhale and exhale, constantly bringing your mind back as it wanders off, is one way, but there are others.

Internally quoting a mantra or even saying it out loud as you sit in quiet solitude can help keep your concentration in the here and now. Traditional mantras, such as Om mani padme hum; om namah shivaya; om shanti om, or even just repeating a long held Ooommmm can focus the mind. Watching the flickering of a candle in front of you is another method. Listening to a guided meditation, particularly in the early stages of becoming used to meditation, is a beneficial way of focusing.

One **guided meditation** I particularly enjoyed was used several times by one yoga teacher. I'm going to set down here my adaptation of it as I can't remember it exactly. It might be as helpful to you as it was to me in relaxing and forgetting the present moment and its worries. I have sometimes found it useful as a tool to help me sleep when my busy mind needs to be quietened.

Sit or lie in a relaxed state. Close your eyes. Now imagine yourself climbing down a circular staircase, down and down and as you go you feel you are leaving your cares and anxieties behind. When you reach the bottom, you find you are in a quiet glen next to a brook. There is a copse of trees beyond the brook. The warm sun is shining and you sit down in the grass and listen to the sounds of the water as it scurries over the stones in the brook. There are birds singing in the trees. You feel a sense of peace from the warm sun, the babbling water and the sound of the birds. After a while, you notice behind you some fields with flowers growing in them. You decide to go and investigate.

There's an open gateway into the first field, which is filled with bluebells. As you enter, you become aware of the scent of the flowers suffused in the warm air and you feel the grass tickling your bare toes as you make your way through the field. The blueness of the flowers gives way to pale yellow as you enter the next field, which is full of primroses. Their delicate fragrance fills your nostrils and the warmth of the ground is absorbed onto the soles of your feet. The third field is a visual delight of pink clover with bees gently buzzing around the delicate heads.

Eventually, after inhaling the scents of the flowers and savoring the beauty of the scenery, you turn back to the stairway and climb it with a sense of peace, relaxed and ready to return to the top. (You can, of course, have your own favorite flowers in the fields to further help relax you).

The traditional Buddhist method of meditation I particularly like to do, though it is difficult when you first start: seated in a comfortable upright position, with eyes closed and concentrating on the breath, follow the breath as it enters your nostrils and is absorbed into the body and then as it is exhaled through your nostrils. Keeping thoughts from taking your concentration away is a challenge. That busy intrusive mind is known as "monkey mind". Science tells us that those sessions of meditation are good for the brain so it's well worth the effort to learn to control the body and mind this way.

Incorporating **mindfulness,** which is basically living in this present moment, into your life will help with the reduction of stress levels. By learning to live in the present, you are helping to overcome the stress of anxiety. Anxiety is a state of mind that is always concerned about something in the future (I heard a good analogy for anxiety: it's like continually holding up an open umbrella in case it rains).

In practicing meditation we become accustomed to trying to be in the here and now, but it can be brought into every aspect of our lives; walking for instance. As we walk, instead of being lost in thought or listening to music via earphones, we can be aware of everything going on around us and of the actions of our body, actually being present rather than somewhere in our heads thinking of something we have to do.

When we eat, if we eat mindfully, savoring each mouthful, we are more aware of having eaten and experienced the enjoyment involved. How many times have you desired a cake or piece of chocolate and have eaten it mindlessly, then thought you could do with another because you weren't really aware of the pleasure of eating the first one. This leads to overeating, which in turn leads to weight gain.

Having said all this about stress and the importance of reducing its impact on the body, there's another way of dealing with it that's being studied by scientists and researchers that has a link to eastern philosophy. Our mindset, or the way we frame things in our minds, can have a bigger effect than trying to get rid of stress. Scientists working on extending the lifespan have acknowledged that stress can be an important factor in our living longer and it's thinking about it in a positive light that helps us to use it beneficially. Research has shown that when people in a study ate healthy food with a negative mindset, they had been primed to think of the food as not enjoyable, then their bodies didn't give positive readings in tests taken afterwards as might be expected after eating wholesome food. So, a negative mindset overrode the benefits of the food. Seeing things in a positive light reduces the risk of stress.

Being happy can predispose you to having long and happy relationships and will help you in your older years. What does "being happy" mean? We can define it as an emotional state characterized by feelings of joy, fulfillment, and satisfaction. Being happy has been found to have positive ramifications for our health. We know from research that happiness can predict health and longevity, but what's involved in acquiring this sense of peace and well-being that underlies a sense of happiness? An established routine that involves self care, e.g. exercising, meditating, a regular and good sleep pattern can lead to a sense of calm and order, which is perhaps necessary for peace and happiness.

Doing the activities that we enjoy are important too: walking in the countryside or forest, taking a luxurious bath, getting absorbed in a good book or film, listening to music, socializing with friends are all ways people find enjoyment. A study found that even just looking at pictures of nature improves our mood. Keeping a journal and writing in it daily, expressing our emotions and recording our personal narrative can help us achieve a positive mindset, which leads to a feeling of happiness.

We also learn from scientific studies that people who are happy don't age as fast as people who are not enjoying life. Perhaps it could be explained by the fact that people who are happier are healthier and feel that they are in control of their lives. They are taking responsibility for how they age, to a certain extent, rather than just letting it happen. Perhaps those who are unhappy are accepting the myths about being older, such as that you should become physically less active, travel less, challenge yourself less. In fact, these beliefs are not true and should be abandoned. If life is to be worth living, it should surely be lived fully at any age.

Is it common for all people to be happier as they age? Apparently it is. It would seem from research carried out into the subject that we do get happier as we get older. Why that should be is mystifying scientists. One study came up with the conclusion that older people are more experienced, so this allows them to deal better with negative emotions like anger and anxiety. Another study concluded that the cause is that older people are more trusting, this leads to health benefits, which leads to happiness.

I recently read some results from a longitudinal study where researchers looked at personality traits to see if they changed as we age. Did people become progressively grumpier as they grew older? Apparently not. The research didn't show any change in basic personality but showed it to be stable over time. Maybe it's just that people are more inclined to voice their dissatisfaction with things as they get older. Change, though, is built into life, and that's what we cover in the next chapter.

6

"Nothing is Permanent, Except Change." *The Buddha*

For a woman, one of the most important events in her life is going through "the change" or "the change of life", as in: "she's going through the change", a euphemism for the **menopause**. The average age for this monumental event is fifty-one. It's a time when she will become no longer fertile, a prospect she will have to learn to come to terms with. Her body will become a stranger to her as the gradually reducing estrogen and progesterone flowing through her system causes never before experienced reactions in various ways, including hot flushes (or flashes, as they say in The States), weight gain, vaginal dryness, dizziness and palpitations, memory problems (brain fog), fatigue and anxiety. Not all women experience all the symptoms and some experience those they do, worse than others.

Longer-term effects can be a reduction in bone density, which is why many older women are susceptible to hip, spine and other bone fractures. Decreased hormone levels can affect the heart in that the arteries become more inflexible, which can affect blood flow. This, combined with weight gain, may be a negative outcome for the heart. It has to be remembered though that it is a natural part of a woman's life cycle and management of the symptoms can be achieved.

A healthy diet with increased calcium, reducing intake of sugar, strength training, exercising for 150 minutes per week, and reducing alcohol are all advisable to the menopausal woman. Giving up smoking is a must (at any age). When I was going through it in my late forties to late fifties, HRT had a poor reputation after being linked to breast cancer in research, so I avoided it. I believe now though, that the research has been discredited or at least HRT is now considered more favorably by some medics as a relief to the symptoms commonly experienced.

You may be prescribed medication by your doctor to ameliorate the symptoms and there are other remedies such as herbal therapies, self-hypnosis, acupuncture, and over-the-counter aids to help with the various effects of the menopause. Every woman experiences it differently, so the way your mother or best friend was affected will differ from your own experience.

The attempts to overcome or live with the effects of the menopause negatively impact those women on a career path by knocking them back or off altogether. Research into this area[8] revealed that ninety-nine percent of women felt that their perimenopausal or menopausal symptoms had a detrimental effect on their careers. Around fifty-nine percent took time off work due to symptoms, and eighteen percent were off for more than eight weeks. Half of the latter resigned or took early retirement. So menopause in the workplace is not adequately supported. Only one in ten female doctors had discussed their symptoms with a manager. Companies are becoming more sympathetic to women going through this life change, but there's still a long way to go.

Recent attempts to get the rights of women going through the menopause covered in law in the UK so that they could be helped through the worst symptoms that have a negative impact on their career have been dismissed by the government. They claim it would discriminate against men. But then aren't women discriminated against by their biology?

"NOTHING IS PERMANENT, EXCEPT CHANGE." THE BUDDHA

The worst symptoms for me were weight gain, a low level of hot flushes, breast cysts - I had seven of them over several years, four in one breast, three in the other; and uterine fibroids. This meant a lot of hospital visits during those years. I had my last cycle aged fifty seven and continue to have breast issues from time to time, even now. Besides the usual multivitamin and glucosamine supplements I was then taking, I added oil of evening primrose to help with the symptoms.

Removal of the breast cysts was carried out by inserting a needle and drawing out the fluid they contained, a process known as aspiration. I noticed during the first six aspirations that the fluid being drawn out was black or dark; it was hard to imagine that in my body. Before the seventh cyst was discovered, I changed my underarm deodorant to a more natural one, omitting any chemicals. The one I decided on was lemon based and yellow. After the discovery of the seventh cyst I went to hospital to have it aspirated and noted with some surprise that the color of the liquid drawn out was green, rather than black or dark. This surely shows a direct link to the chemicals we put in our bodies via deodorant. I've always used a natural one ever since.

"NOTHING IS PERMANENT, EXCEPT CHANGE." THE BUDDHA

So how should we feel about this big change in our life? We might mourn the loss of fertility even though we no longer want to have children; after menopause, though, we no longer have the choice. The prospect of ceasing to be considered a target for the male gaze may be another. But we might also appreciate the cessation of the monthly menses and all that it entails, as well as the worry about pregnancy, as positives. We might experience a new sense of independence, of moving into a new chapter of our life and, with it, the anticipation of new possibilities.

For men, apparently, the equivalent of the female menopause is the **andropause**. However, it is not the same in that there is no sudden drop in hormone level, as when, for women, they cease menstruation. Men experience a gradual reduction in testosterone from around their thirties and few symptoms can be attributed to it. They may experience a midlife crisis when they believe that they have reached the halfway stage of their life and have not achieved all that they had hoped to. This can lead to anxiety and depression, which a visit to a doctor or counselor can help with[9].

"NOTHING IS PERMANENT, EXCEPT CHANGE." THE BUDDHA

Changing the way we look because we're aging is not compulsory. If we have always liked to give a nod to the latest fashion, why shouldn't we continue to do so? My mother's generation seemed to wear clothes "appropriate" for their age, which was part of the image society constructed for older women, who were subtly told to wear their dresses well below the knees (when the fashion was for above the knee), legs to be covered by wearing tights (American Tan being a popular color) in all weathers and hair to be worn short. Thank goodness that doesn't apply anymore - we can wear pretty much what we want if, and when, we want to. The disapprovers will still show their annoyance at your not following the well-worn path, but we are becoming inured to the criticism as more people challenge the status quo about aging.

Managing the changes in our appearance as we age is important if we have always taken an interest in how we look. What clothes we wear, how we wear our hair and what we put on our skin may change over time to accommodate our maturing bodies. If you've always liked to dress with a nod to the latest fashion, then there's no reason that should change as you grow older.

"NOTHING IS PERMANENT, EXCEPT CHANGE." THE BUDDHA

If **fashion** is what we buy, style is what we make it. We choose clothes according to our chosen style. I like a classic style with a modern look; natural fibers where possible. They do wash and wear longer than human-made fibers, but I wondered, in this time of climate change awareness, which were best for the environment, so I did some research into the subject. It seemed to suggest that both natural and human made fibers have a negative impact on the environment, but natural fibers may be best, especially if you recycle them and buy them secondhand, or pre-loved, as they are now termed. There is a burgeoning trend in secondhand clothes, and that is obviously a good thing for the environment as well as people's pockets; not so good for the fashion industry, maybe.

Style is how we present our own individuality - our own way of doing things, of expressing ourselves through what we wear, of how we interpret fashion. It's said that you either have it or you don't. But who is to say? Who is to judge? Are there style police out there? Certainly, we can read articles in magazines on how to achieve it, informing us that if we are a certain age, we shouldn't wear this or have our hair like that. But then if we slavishly followed rules, we'd lose our individuality - OUR style. As we grow older, we get to know ourselves better and our style develops along with us.

Now I'm in my seventies and have stopped highlighting my hair and trying to hide the grey. There were several reasons I chose this path: it would be healthier as no more chemicals would be absorbed through my scalp, it would save time at the hairdressers, it would be part of the self acceptance of "me" in the newfound confidence maturity was instilling in me and of course, it would save money. I'm also growing it long again. We women are usually told in magazines that after fifty we should wear our hair shorter and certainly over sixty, we should not wear it long. There are many women today bucking that trend and becoming good examples of what aging in the twenty-first centuries should be. I'm joining them. That's not to say that every woman will want to grow their hair long in their older years, but the choice should be there without criticism from the self-appointed style police.

A couple of years ago, a friend and I were discussing clothes. She told me about the new top her husband had bought her for her birthday recently from "that shop up the hill, you know the one - it's for people of our age". It really surprised her to learn that I never buy clothes from 'age appropriate' shops. I told her I buy my clothes from the usual high street shops or online, even charity shops and eBay. It just doesn't occur to me to look at clothes that other people think are suitable for me because of my age. I think I changed my friend's attitude towards clothes shopping.

Skin care is a huge money spinner for beauty product companies and anti-aging products are massively popular. I first created a skin care routine for myself when I was sixteen after being invited to a beauty product "party". From then on I was hooked and have always looked after my skin; cleansing it with baby lotion, then closing the pores with toner and applying day or night cream, whichever is relevant.

Serum has become a recent addition to this skin care regime. It's usually sold in a small bottle with a dropper and is an intensified concoction of hyaluronic acid or retinol and other ingredients of which only a few drops need to be applied nightly (or daily) to get the desired results. There's also the exfoliating face wash once or twice a week and a face mask to close the pores. A good sun protecting cream worn on the face is a daily necessity if going out, regardless of weather. Men, too, today are encouraged to take care of their skin and there is a huge choice of products designed especially for them.

So many anti-aging products are on the market now because women want to push back time and keep their youthful looks. The media are a driver in this, urging women overtly or often subliminally to dress this way, behave that way, above all - look youthful. New facial treatments can now be purchased at your local beauticians: micro-dermabrasion, chemical peels, micro-needling, laser skin rejuvenation etc. Hollywood stars appear on screen and in magazines, their expressionless faces taut with botox or a facelift, lips injected to plump them up, character smoothed out along with the lines and wrinkles. I've watched some of them in amazement, wondering why they don't understand how their lips, for instance, look just plain weird. Obviously, they are following the latest trend and wanting to "improve" their looks, sadly, not succeeding in most cases.

Of course, I can understand that when we feel young inside, we don't want to catch sight of ourselves in a mirror and see a reflection that doesn't fit with the way we feel we should look. It happens to me all the time! However, I'm happy to let nature take its course, aided by creams and lotions, etc.

Once we are into the age society considers old, we will experience changes that happen naturally, such as deterioration in our senses, we might need new glasses and perhaps hearing aids will be in order, we may become a little more forgetful, gum disease could become a problem for us and our teeth will most likely present problems. Having regular medical checkups will alert us to any developing issues and looking after our bodies with a good diet, regular exercise, sufficient quality sleep and keeping in touch with friends and family will all help us cope with the changes.

Studies show that no matter what age you take up a healthier way of living, you will make a positive difference to your life and add to your longevity. Just by making a few lifestyle changes you can improve your health and, therefore, the quality of your life. Becoming active, eating less but healthier food, sleeping well, being creative, developing and

"NOTHING IS PERMANENT, EXCEPT CHANGE." THE BUDDHA

maintaining a social network of friends and family and becoming involved in your community, perhaps by volunteering, are all ways to be in some control of your aging and to live a healthier and fuller life.

Conclusion

As I stated in Chapter 1 of this book, over thirty years ago I made changes to my lifestyle affecting diet and exercise that I've retained and which have stood me in good stead when it comes to my health and aging well. So, I've reached this stage of my life having dealt with inherited health issues - the pre-diabetes which was a warning that I managed to overcome and ocular hypertension, a pre-glaucoma condition which is being kept in check with eye drops. Don't forget we are told that genes account for only twenty percent of health outcomes, our own efforts make up the other eighty percent. Other than that, I am in good shape and so I wanted to share my journey and the research findings that I've put into practice to, hopefully, be of use to or inspire others.

Thinking yourself younger than your chronological age, setting yourself a goal way into the future to encourage you to think positively and to live in the now without anxiety, keeping yourself flexible so that you can bend down easier and retaining a sense of balance to prevent yourself from falling, as well as eating healthily are all validated by re-

CONCLUSION

search studies to help us as we age. The importance of mindset in this process is vital.

As I state in Chapter 2, I intend to live another twenty years at least. I may not achieve that, of course, and the unraveling of my genes as I go deeper into older age may bring more unpleasant surprises that negatively affect my life. However, staying positive is beneficial to health, so I shall continue to refuse to accept the stereotypical older woman image and carry on being the ageless person I see myself as, moving freely, thinking clearly, interacting with family and friends and caring about society and the world we live in. Oh, and treating life like an adventure.

I hope you have found much in these pages to be of help to you in your own experience of growing older, whatever age you may be now and I wish you well in your endeavors to live a long, healthy and fulfilled life.

NB *It's best to talk to your doctor before making any major changes to your lifestyle regarding diet and exercise, particularly if you have an underlying health condition.*

References

[9]Androniki Naska, PhD; Eleni Oikonomou, BS; Antonia Trichopoulou, MD; et al: *Siesta in Healthy Adults and Coronary Mortality in the General Population.* Arch Intern Med. 2007;167(3):296-301. doi:10.1001/archinte.167.3.296

[2]Buettner, Dan. 2012 *The Blue Zones 9 Lessons for Living Longer.* Washington DC: National Geographic.

[12]Huberman Lab: Dr. Alia Crum: Science of Mindsets for Health & Performance: Jan 24 2022.

[6]https://www.ons.gov.uk/census

[3]Journal of the American Heart Association Report: Older women who ate more plant-based protein had lower risk of premature dementia-related death. Feb 24 2021

[4]I-Min Lee, MBBS, ScD1,2; Eric J. Shiroma, ScD3; Masamitsu Kamada, PhD4; et al: Association of Step Volume and Intensity With All-Cause Mortality in Older Women: JAMA Intern Med. 2019;179(8):1105-1112. doi:10.1001/jamainternmed.2019.0899

[1]Pyrkov, T.V., Avchaciov, K., Tarkhov, A.E. et al. Longitudinal analysis of blood markers reveals progressive loss of resilience and predicts human lifespan limit. *Nat Commun* 12, 2765 (2021). https://doi.org/10.1038/s41467-021-23014-1

REFERENCES

[8]Newson, Dr Louise of Newson Health Research and Education. 2021

[9]NHS website: www.nhs.uk

[10]"Feeling Young Could Mean Your Brain is Aging More Slowly." NeuroscienceNews. 3 July 2018 https://neurosciencenews.com/feeling-young-brain-aging-9504

[5]Peter Elwood, Julieta Galante, Janet Pickering, Stephen Palmer, Antony Bayer, Yoav Ben-Shlomo, Marcus Longley, John Gallacher *Healthy Lifestyles Reduce the Incidence of Chronic Diseases and Dementia: Evidence from the Caerphilly Cohort Study: Published: December 9,2013*

[12]https://www.sleepfoundation.org/physical-health/how-sleep-affects-immunity

Acknowledgements

I acknowledge with gratitude the following people for their invaluable help with this book:

Alpha Reader and Sounding Board: Trevor Innes

Beta Reader: Jules Burdett (julesdoesyoga.com)

Beta Reader: Paul Lanigan

Beta Reader: Margaret Shaw

I also want to acknowledge my close friend, Seonaid Wootton, who Beta read and proofread the first incarnation of this book and was a great support in the project; other close friends, Cliona Woods and Rosemary Andrews, and my son, Dom Gifford were Beta Readers in that first incarnation and provided useful feedback. Dom was a huge help in the formatting of the book for publication.

I'm grateful to them all for their help and support.

About the Author

Patricia A Cusack is an artist and writer. She has written short stories for adults and created books for children. This is the first nonfiction book which Patricia has published. She has an Honors degree in Psychology & Social Policy, having always been interested in people. For fourteen years she was a volunteer counselor for a charity for women. Patricia lives in the UK and finds inspiration for her work from tradition and innovation. For many years, she ran her own business selling secondhand books, specializing in classic literature and illustrated books, sought out by her then husband. She's always enjoyed writing in one form or another.

Further Books in this series:

Book 2: **Healthy Aging Tips: Discovering Yourself** (working title) will be launched in a few months' time. In this book I will be looking at how we can find who we were meant to be before we built up childhood defenses as we aged, through psychology and philosophy. Also, our place in our family tree through genealogy, and how we are affected by our inherited genes.

ABOUT THE AUTHOR

I spent six years and more researching my family tree and I will tell you how I did it and how I solved the mystery of my great-grandfather's "murder"; my mother had told me that her maternal grandfather was killed unlawfully before she was born and didn't know how, why or where. My searches answered all these questions.

If you are interested in receiving updates and eventual launch date for future books please go to my website and leave your email address for me to contact you. I can also be found on Instagram: @patricia.cusack.author. I have an author page on Amazon where details of other books I've created or written will be displayed.

Thank You

Now that you've reached the end of the book, I want to thank you for reading it.

I'd like to get the information it contains out to as many people as possible. If you found this book helpful, I would greatly appreciate you leaving me a review. This will help others find the book.

Printed in Great Britain
by Amazon